We Are Gatekeepers

A Self-Reflective Leadership Challenge for Nurses at all Levels

Jaimee L. Gerrie

Ideas into Books® WESTVIEW

Kingston Springs, Tennessee 37082

Ideas into Books®
W E S T V I E W
P.O. Box 605
Kingston Springs, TN 37082
www.publishedbywestview.com

ISBN 978-1-62880-093-7

First edition, January 2016

Printed in the United States of America on acid free paper.

This book is dedicated to all of the nurses that make up our profession.

With sincere gratitude and appreciation I would like to say:

Thank you to my husband and children
for their endless love and support.

Thank you to my mentor and friend
Erie Chapman MTS, JD
for his support and encouragement.

Thank you to my editor and friend
Janice Repka JD, MA, MFA
for her time, expertise, and guidance.

Thank you to my colleague and friend
Kathleen Pawlanta RN, MSN, NP
for her peer review and encouragement.

Thank you to my dear friend
Julie Wiater BBA, PHR
for encouraging me to reach beyond
my comfort zone.

Contents

Introduction

Thank you for choosing *We Are Gatekeepers*.

The writing of this book was stimulated by my passion for nursing, the nursing profession, and the desire to promote a healthy nursing culture that is safe for every patient. I have been a Registered Nurse for over 20 years. I earned my Masters of Science in Nursing Degree with an emphasis in Nursing Management and Leadership from Walden University and I am ANCC Board Certified in Medical Surgical Nursing. I am employed as an Assistant Professor in the School of Nursing at Lake Superior State University.

Over the past two decades I have served in practice as a staff nurse, a nurse leader, and a nurse manager. I am the founder and owner of UPvision Consulting, LLC. Through this business I serve as a nurse and health care consultant promoting positive outcomes for nurses and patients.

I believe it is necessary for nurses at all levels to periodically perform a self-assessment and get back to the fundamentals of nursing and why they became a nurse. It is also my belief that nurses entering practice need to be guided through the bridging of education and practice. I believe this because over the past 20 years I have observed nurses being challenged with the temptation to practice outside of the Professional Scopes and Standards of Practice and Code of Ethics for Nursing. This challenge is concerning because in every decision and action taken outside of these standards, patients, nurses, and organizations are placed at risk for harm.

The chapters that lie before you will lead you on a motivational journey to self-discovery. The pages are designed to read as slowly or quickly as you like. You may move through the book in order or take the time to reflect on different topics in order of your interest. Each chapter will present you with a self-reflective challenge and opportunity to reflect on your own practice, to recognize the challenges you face in maintaining your Professional Scopes and Standards of Practice, and to claim or re-claim your own practice as a professional nurse.

The professional oath every nurse takes upon graduation from nursing school is a reminder of the responsibility each nurse has to practice with integrity. Nurses have a duty to instill trust as competent, knowledgeable, independent, and collaborative members of the health care team. Entering into and serving in practice as leaders, guiding, directing, and managing health care is our job. Nurses at every level must allow this oath and commitment to resonate in and to positively influence their behavior in professional practice on a consistent and unwavering basis. Nurses must clearly understand the role of the professional nurse, and the impact this role has in health care. As the gatekeeper it is each and every nurse that must create this understanding through the demonstration of professional practice.

The term gatekeeper is chosen in the title and utilized repetitively throughout this book in reference to the professional nurse. It is used to serve as a reminder that nurses are not passive in their work. Nurses have a responsibility to guard and protect those in their care. Nurses are responsible to assure the gates to health care are open and welcoming to all who are in need. Nurses must help others navigate the health care environment. Nurses serve through advocacy, experience, and education. The term gatekeeper is strong and helps to create the image of nursing, communicating to others that nurses are both independent and collaborative in their role within the health care team.

Although it is most universally recognized that the professional nurse is a four-year degree nurse, nurses at all levels can benefit from the message of this book. Nurses at all levels are engaged in the care of the lives of others, serve as advocates, and hold the responsibility to uphold Standards of Practice and Code of Ethics within the scope of their degree level and practice.

I welcome you now to begin. I am hopeful that you will find as much enjoyment and passion in the reading of this book as I have had in the writing of it. Each chapter will end with a challenge. This challenge is repetitive and unfolds as it repeats. I encourage you to reflect on how these words will inspire you in your journey as a gatekeeper and your responsibility to engage collectively and professionally to lead the future of health care.

Gatekeepers Own Who We Are

As gatekeepers we are called to own who we are. This means that we must recognize and accept that we are nurses. This is not different from accepting responsibility and embracing our power, however, this sense of ownership for our image as a profession has traditionally lacked in demonstration. This can be noted in the many definitions or visions of what a nurse is and what a nurse does.

Let's take a moment to address history in nursing and bring some insight to the above statement. The history of nursing demonstrates a perpetual lack of ownership in nursing. The early nursing practice creates a vision of nurses from the field with no formal education, to a hospital setting where nurses were educated through clinical practice (Selanders & Patrick, 2012). This transition has positive significance in the development of education, quality, and standards of practice. It places the nurse, however, in the role of dependency in this practice. Nurses became dependent on the organization to provide them with an income and on physicians to guide and direct nursing care. This hierarchal structure, push for conformity and loss of independent thinking created a culture of co-dependency in nursing that undermines our progression yet today (Lynaugh, 2008). This can be observed in organizations that continue delivery of care under a medical model. Modern day efforts to improve outcomes in health care delivery rely on non-nurse led programs to script language for nursing at the bedside and to require conformity to standardization or measures for achieving standards of care.

Although individual nurses have taken the lead, for example, by obtaining advanced degrees, serving in administrative positions, performing research, being activists for change, in our profession throughout history and today, the mindset that nursing is an independent yet collaborative profession struggles to exist within the ranks of the nursing profession and health care as a whole. You may agree or disagree with this statement. However, think about the image of the nurse. For many, the first image that comes to mind is the guardian angel. Nurses often choose to wear them on their name tags or scrubs as a gift from a patient or a loved one. Visualize the caring hands. These hands provide a gentle reminder of our role to provide a healing touch. Consider the lady with the lamp as an image of strength and endless love for the wounded. These images present a strong presence, one of support, comforting, and willingness to take on another's suffering as our own in a higher calling. These are images we send to our community.

If we own who we are in the image of the nurse it is important to recognize that in the soft images we demonstrate, our full image is often hidden. I was recently at a graduation event for one of my son's good friends. I was talking with another mother and she asked me if I was still a nurse? I replied, "Of course" as I could not imagine being anything else. She responded quickly with "Oh, I did not know that a nurse could be a teacher. I thought you now worked at the University instead of in a hospital." Our conversation evolved into a discussion about what it means to be a nurse and the many roles and responsibilities nurses have. This mother visualized nurses as servants providing comfort and support at the bedside in times of illness, yet did not relate that nurses are strong and powerful advocates and serve in many other roles as well, such as educators, lawyers, business owners, and so much more.

The above anecdote demonstrates the struggle nurses have with taking ownership of who we are and what we do. Without the demonstration and communication of this ownership our image is only partially presented which creates a vision that fails to include autonomy, power, responsibility, and accountability. Nurses present an image then that devalues our role and the uniqueness of our profession. When this occurs in a health care setting nurses risk opening the doors for patients to experience greater suffering. Presentation of only the soft image of the nurse misleads others and can and often does result in standardization verses individualization of care. Often other health care and non-health care professionals step in to direct and control our practice without understanding and respect for our knowledge, Scopes and Standards of Practice, and professional ethics. Reflecting back to the anecdote, nurses are then seen as servants and the risk is that our practice is controlled and directed by other professionals.

Gatekeepers before Us

Nursing is supported in history by some very influential nurses, such as Florence Nightingale, Virginia Henderson, and Mildred Tuttle. It is necessary to pay respect for their work and to bring attention to them for their willingness to own who they were, accept responsibility, have courage, take risks, educate, develop others, and push for safe and independent practice regardless of perceived or actual barriers in their professional practice. These nurses were gatekeepers. They did not role-model a co-dependent professional nursing practice. They role modeled their acceptance and ownership of their nursing practice.

Florence Nightingale, in her views on nursing as a profession, advocates that nursing is an independent profession focused on collaboration with other health care professionals in the management of health care (Selanders & Patrick, 2012). The reluctance of some nurses today to take this same level of ownership has led to the creation of only soft images of the profession. Although these soft images when practiced provide those we serve with empathy and compassion, the failure to communicate in this same practice that we are tough advocates and managers of patient care misguides the professional relationships nurses are responsible to develop and maintain. It has prevented nurses from not just communicating value as the gatekeeper in health care, but from consistently demonstrating it as well.

A Vision of Ownership

At this time, create a visual picture in your mind of the person in your life that if you lost would leave you to feel most devastated. Picture this person becoming ill. As this person begins his or her journey into the environment of health care you are unable to be by his or her side. This person will be greeted by a nurse, a gatekeeper for his or her care.

What kind of gatekeeper do you visualize?

What role does this gatekeeper serve?

How does this gatekeeper behave?

Now, reflect on this image. Did you envision a nurse role modeling after Florence Nightingale or any other leader in our profession's history?

It has been suggested that because it is the side of nursing that is most communicated that most would picture a gatekeeper that is kind, caring, and compassionate. Most would visualize a gatekeeper that would care for their loved ones as their own, a guardian angel, with gentle hands, or the lady with the lamp. When I presented this scenario to a group of sophomore nursing students they also visualized a gatekeeper that was knowledgeable, an advocate, focused on quality, prepared, positive, realistic, responsible, and never willing to sacrifice standard of care.

Take a moment now to reflect on your own practice and your vision.

Do you picture yourself as the gatekeeper in your vision?

If you do are you being honest?

Do you role model these traits and qualities consistently with every human to human encounter?

Do you consistently demonstrate and communicate an image of ownership for your role as a gatekeeper?

Self-reflection is not always easy. It requires honesty, integrity, and openness. It requires a willingness to accept our imperfections. If you are not the gatekeeper in your vision, do not spend time asking yourself why. We want to avoid practicing as co-dependent nurses. We must not point fingers at others, place blame on environments, or what is not present in our work that lend to the challenge of not communicating or demonstrating our full image, of not being prepared, responsible, accountable, and less attentive to standard of care. Choosing to walk a path of co-dependency verses taking ownership of our image decreases our value as an individual nurse and as a profession. This is how our power is lost to other non-nursing professionals and our ability to govern our own profession is forfeited. What is most important in this moment is that you, as a strong independent and collaborative nursing professional, begin to accept ownership of your role as a gatekeeper and actively make changes to turn your weaknesses, such as lack of confidence, lack of assertiveness, or whatever you identified in your vision into strengths.

Reflect on your vision. Commit to accepting ownership of your image. What matters most is that as a nurse you own who you are in the full image of the nurse and that you make the changes necessary to do so. It is important to demonstrate and communicate your image as gatekeeper and role model demonstrating self-respect and authority for your professional practice. Don't give your power away by hiding in an image of caring without accepting the responsibility of what that caring means. In the image of the caring professional you are strong and serve as an independent yet collaborative member of the health care team. You serve as the gatekeeper assuring that those we serve receive compassionate and quality care.

Using Ownership to Teach Others

I will never forget my first medication error as a new nurse. Excited to take the leap into practice, I immediately set aside my learned standards of practice and delivered a medication to the wrong patient. I was working my first two shifts as a novice nurse. On the first day I was assigned thirteen patients for medication administration. I accomplished this without difficulty, gaining confidence in my skills, and assuring that I followed all standards of medication administration which at that time were known as the five rights. These are Right patient, Right drug, Right dose, Right time, and Right route. On the second day I gained one more patient to my assignment. This patient was an elderly woman who had been admitted with dementia. I prepared for medication administration the same as I did the day before and set forth with confidence that all would go well. I approached my first patient room. This was the room of the new patient I acquired. I pulled out the medication drawer, found the patient medication administration record, followed the rights of medication administration while I prepared this patients morning cardiac medications. I entered the room and noted that the patient was not wearing an arm band. At this in-pass, I failed to serve in my caring role as a patient advocate and a nurse that maintained the professional standards of care. Because I felt confident that I had performed the rights of medication administration I also felt confident this was the correct person and I administered the medication. It was not until I resumed my medication pass a few minutes later that I realized I moved ahead by one room and gave a non-cardiac patient another patients cardiac medication. Now as you can imagine if you have ever made a medication error I felt incredibly small. I was worried and scared and embarrassed in my lack of competent and safe practice. I immediately responded however by notifying my preceptor, contacting the physician, and taking full ownership for my failure. The patient did not suffer any negative outcomes from this mistake. I have never forgotten my first medication error and as a result have never made another one.

While lecturing to a group of novice nursing students about medication administration safety, I shared this experience and all the details making strong reference to our professional responsibilities of our nursing profession, which is to practice and uphold the highest standard of care. Solidifying my message with this example and stressing that my failure to uphold the highest standard of care, led to a passionate moment in encouraging students to learn from my mistakes verses their own. I connected these students with the opportunity I had to humble myself in this experience and in my professional practice, to open myself to a realization that as a gatekeeper I must own my image and communicate and demonstrate who I am as a professional nurse, and regardless of the situation, a failure to practice at or above standard is never acceptable.

As I brought my story to an end, one student broke the intensity and called out "that's it professor, just own it!" In that second we all laughed. Little did this student know what a teaching tool that this statement that brought about so much laughter would become that semester. Each time a student was faced with a challenge regarding the maintaining of our professional standards of care someone would use those words "just own it!" providing that student with a reminder and giving them the confidence to assure that they choose to do what is right verses knowing what is right and choosing a different path placing a patient at risk of harm. This phrase was used to help students learn the importance of demonstrating as well as communicating the full image of the nurse.

Spending time in reflection since that semester I have come to realize that this statement so innocently made brings clarity to the frustrations I have had since my own failure to uphold a standard of practice. This frustration is the passivity or lack of "just owning it" within individual nursing practice and our profession as a whole that lends to an explanation as to why gatekeepers in general look to others outside of nursing to solve nursing issues in health care, such as medication safety, patient to nurse ratios, safe staffing, and so much more.

Gatekeepers create a vision for others of the soft image in nursing care by limiting themselves or allowing themselves to be defined by the tasks they perform verses their duty to the profession. This often leads to a failure to take ownership for who they are as a nursing professional and the gatekeepers they are.

In ending this chapter I leave you with a challenge.

Understand that as nurses our profession is only governed by nurses. We have the responsibility to practice nursing with full authority within our independent as well as collaborative and delegated roles according to our scopes and standards of professional practice. As nurses, we have the obligation to *own* who we are, to serve as *gatekeepers*, with the authority to advocate, change health care environments, delegate, develop and implement policy, design and direct delivery of care, communicate and role model our professional duty, upholding the highest standard in quality and service to others.

Chapter One Self-Reflection Challenges

There are many desired qualities and traits of a professional nurse that demonstrate and communicate ownership of our image. These include but are not limited to: integrity, compassionate, advocate, responsible, knowledgeable. Reflecting back on your chapter reading what qualities as a professional nurse would you like to strengthen?

_____

_____

_____

_____

_____

_____

_____

_____

_____

_____

_____

_____

_____

_____

_____

Reflecting on the qualities and traits you wish to strengthen as a nurse what three things can you do immediately to begin to strengthen them and communicate and demonstrate ownership for your image as a nurse?

_____

_____

_____

_____

_____

_____

_____

_____

_____

_____

_____

_____

_____

_____

_____

Develop or outline a plan, including dates, to achieve these three things.

_____

_____

_____

_____

_____

_____

_____

_____

_____

_____

_____

_____

_____

_____

_____

_____

_____

_____

How will the achievement of your plan demonstrate you have accepted ownership for who you are both as a professional nurse individually and within the nursing profession?

_____

_____

_____

_____

_____

_____

_____

_____

_____

_____

_____

_____

_____

_____

_____

_____

Gatekeepers Accept Responsibility

As gatekeepers, we must accept responsibility. We have responsibility to our profession and to role model our independent authority in our nursing practice. If we think about who governs our practice then it must be understood that those in positions outside of the nursing profession, such as unions, non-nurse administrators, legislators, and other health care professionals do not hold the authority to control or direct our practice within our boundaries and scopes and standards of care or span of control.

Mary Koloroutis (2004) discusses professional nursing stating that "responsibility, authority and accountability for professional nursing practice are determined based on licensure and nurse practice acts, educational preparation and experience, professional standards, regulatory standards, and position descriptions within an organization." She also notes that "it is important for nurses and all other members of the health care team to understand and articulate their boundaries based on their practice discipline and their individual level of knowledge and skills."

It is the responsibility of the gatekeeper to communicate and demonstrate what expectations need to be held by the profession. This is done by accepting the responsibility to be proactive in the environment in which we work, our profession as a whole, and by helping those outside of the nursing profession to understand how to support the profession of nursing without giving away the ownership of the control or direction of nursing practice.

A Vision for Accepting Responsibility

Consider the nurses or colleagues who create stress within an environment by not accepting the responsibility to practice safely, by complaining about their work, or by gossiping and criticizing others in their work. As a gatekeeper who is proactive and accepting of our professional responsibility, this behavior must be addressed. If the behavior does not change, then there is a responsibility for the chain of command to be followed in dealing with this careless and inappropriate nurse. As the gatekeeper we must not relinquish that responsibility to another or ignore the behavior. Tolerance of negative attitude and behavior creates a negative environment that often results in low morale, conflict within a nursing team, and decrease in nursing satisfaction. This leads to higher rates of nursing turnover, increased errors in patient care, and a stressed nursing care environment, jeopardizing patient safety. As a gatekeeper it is our responsibility to protect our patients and to keep them safe in our care.

Gatekeepers also learn their professional scopes and standards of practice and help other professionals learn them as well. By communicating and demonstrating these standards through application consistently in practice. For example, gatekeepers must accept the responsibility to accept or deny the performance of any delegated task of the physician based on their professional scopes and standards of practice, code of ethics, and the foreseen outcome of that delegated task.

Refusing to Play the Blame Game

Gatekeepers have more than an obligation to understand and articulate boundaries in care.

Gatekeepers have the responsibility to maintain ownership of them and to carry them out as role models for others. Gatekeepers have a responsibility to collaborate with respect to the boundaries of other professionals and assure that those same professionals support and view nursing as respected partners in health care.

To do this, every gatekeeper must avoid placing blame on others for the failures in nursing practice related to the delivery of care and professional growth. Every gatekeeper must also not expect others outside of the nursing profession to manage the profession's failure to accept responsibility in the professional setting.

Gatekeepers must take the responsibility to accept the authority to practice independently within the scopes and standards of their professional nursing licensure and education. In a discussion regarding partnerships in re-designing health care, Chard (2013), states that nurses can practice as full partners with other health care providers as long as organizations support the creation of an environment that promotes this partnership. Many might agree. We must understand that when the word organization is used, it means all professionals and employees within that environment. Unfortunately, the fact that we as gatekeepers need to look for an organization to promote this environment demonstrates that we have not already accepted the responsibility to practice with full authority within that organization. We have allowed ourselves individually as professionals and collectively as a profession to be regarded without value for our independent and collaborative roles.

In chapter one, I referenced Lynaugh, 2008 noting the historical perspective of nursing in which nurses are placed in the role of dependency resulting in a loss of independence and co-dependent nursing practice. I made reference to modern day efforts to improve outcomes in health care delivery, rely on non-nurse led programs to script language for nursing at the bedside and to require conformity to standardization or measures for achieving standards of care. Many nurses have experienced these efforts in their organization. Certainly, at some point it has been asked "why am I being told what to say and how to say it to my patients?" Gatekeepers have questions why nursing care is being molded for quality assurance without attention to individualization of that care.

Why are others governing over nursing practice and directing it in this way? Shouldn't nurses and other health care professionals alike already be performing in practice to such a high standard that these things should not be needed?

The answer to this question is *absolutely!* Unfortunately, these programs and mandates have become a reality because standards of care have not been upheld by each and every practitioner. In nursing this is a demonstration of gatekeepers not accepting the responsibility to practice according to standard and a failure to own their role with each and every encounter and action in practice.

Taking Personal Responsibility as a Gatekeeper

I am hopeful you are focusing internally at this time and thinking about your own practice and the responsibility you have taken as a gatekeeper in your organization. Take a moment to reflect on your thoughts. Visualize how you have demonstrated this responsibility. If you are seeing that you have not yet accepted full responsibility as a gatekeeper, take time to reflect on the ways in which you can begin. Identify that as a nurse you have the authority to claim this responsibility. It is not dependent as Chard (2013) noted on whether or not the organization is supportive of an environment that recognizes the gatekeeper as a full partner in health care. This has only become an obstacle that gatekeepers as a profession have allowed to develop. It can be overcome.

Understand that in the creation of the image of nursing, each demonstration of the acceptance of responsibility is caring. Through the consistent willingness to practice as a responsible gatekeeper we go beyond the limited image of caring that we historically created for our profession and we gain control over what we are licensed and educated to do.

Creating Opportunity to Accept Responsibility

When interviewing gatekeepers for positions of employment, there is a favorite question I like to ask. The question is: "If you could create the environment you come to work in everyday, what would it look like to you?" During follow up evaluations throughout a gatekeeper's employment, I like to bring this question back and ask: "Does the environment you work in everyday look like the one you would create? If yes, how? If no, why not?" then I ask, "What responsibility have you accepted in creating the environment you desire to work in every day? If none, what responsibility can you begin to accept?"

I have found that gatekeepers often become quiet with this line of questioning. Those that answer with confidence almost consistently comment that the environment would be neat and clean, that teamwork is displayed, that gatekeepers receive support from management, nurse to patient ratios are safe, or that work schedules are stable for work life balance. When asked what responsibility the gatekeeper takes into practice to create this environment, however, the responses often demonstrate a lack of understanding for the role of the professional nurse in health care in regard to responsibility.

Answers range from the need for other gatekeepers to change negative behavior, or for administrations to place nursing environments and beside care above monetary needs, and compensation for service. Gatekeepers have made statements like these: "If management would hold others accountable and follow up on issues, then the environment would be a good one," or "If the State would pass nurse-to-patient ratios and mandate how many patients nurses care for, then management would have to listen and the environment would be better."

Most gatekeepers would agree that nurse managers need to accept responsibility as much as any gatekeeper, and assure resources are provided to promote safe environments. It is with great hope that regardless of the level of service of any gatekeeper, this book will spark reflection on practice and become a catalyst for strengthening the role of the professional nurse.

Questions like the ones in the above example are asked to encourage nurses to begin to understand that without an acceptance of responsibility at all levels to act and practice like the professional they studied to become, control over professional practice will likely continue to be given away. The risk is that nursing will continue to hide in an image that demonstrates only the "soft stuff" in health care verses serving as the leaders we are.

The risk is that, generations of gatekeepers will continue to practice in a fragmented, chaotic, misguided and self-focused manner. This will continue to promote an ongoing loss of quality, advocacy, respect for decision making, and power as a collaborative, and independent partner in the management of care.

Remembering the Role of the Gatekeeper to Serve

In a book titled *Crying is Not an Option*, Borkowksi (2012) demonstrates an effort to empower family as caregiver to advocate endlessly for their loved ones. She recognized the challenges of health care and witnessed the failure of gatekeepers to accept responsibility in the care of her spouse. Helping caregivers and patients advocate for themselves in health care is a good thing. It prevents errors and poor care from occurring. It places patients and families in control of their own care. What is not acceptable is that this advice is given as a result of the gatekeeper's lack of responsibility to assure this care is already excellent. If every gatekeeper independently and collaboratively accepted the responsibility to care appropriately, quality of care would not be in question, advocacy would be collaborative with families and patients rather than combative and forceful, and respect for decision making as a partner in health care would be present.

Gatekeepers are responsible to determine what is appropriate for the safe delivery of care in each care environment. Gatekeepers are responsible to determine what resources are available for that delivery of care and to develop nursing care delivery systems and models that utilize these resources efficiently. Each organization has its own personality, its own barriers to resources, and the care in each environment will be delivered in a different way.

The gatekeeper must accept the responsibility to not add to the suffering of patients and families by forcing them to advocate for what should automatically be delivered at their time of need. The gatekeeper must role model the acceptance of this responsibility consistently and become the expert and respected collaborative voice at the table in regard to nursing care delivery.

In ending of this chapter I leave you with a challenge.

Understand that as nurses our profession is only governed by nurses. We have the *responsibility* to practice nursing with full authority within our independent as well as collaborative and delegated roles according to our scopes and standards of professional practice. As nurses, we have the obligation to *own* who we are, to serve as *gatekeepers*, with the authority to advocate, change health care environments, delegate, develop and implement policy, design and direct delivery of care, communicate and role model our professional duty, upholding the highest standard in quality and service to others.

Chapter Two Self-Reflection Challenges

Reflect on a time where you truly accepted responsibility as a gatekeeper in the care of others.

_____

_____

_____

_____

_____

_____

_____

_____

_____

_____

_____

_____

_____

_____

_____

_____

_____

_____

Describe the outcome of this experience.

_____

_____

_____

_____

_____

_____

_____

_____

_____

_____

_____

_____

_____

_____

_____

_____

_____

_____

Reflect on a time where you did not accept the responsibility of your role as gatekeeper in the care of others as much as you could have.

_____

_____

_____

_____

_____

_____

_____

_____

_____

_____

_____

_____

_____

_____

_____

_____

_____

_____

Discuss why you believe you did not accept this responsibility as much as you could have.

_____

_____

_____

_____

_____

_____

_____

_____

_____

_____

_____

_____

_____

_____

_____

_____

_____

_____

If you had the opportunity to experience this situation again, what would you do differently?

_____

_____

_____

_____

_____

_____

_____

_____

_____

_____

_____

_____

_____

_____

_____

_____

_____

_____

_____

Gatekeepers are Accountable

As gatekeepers we must be accountable and to be accountable, we must accept responsibility. Accountability is not punishment. It is not the action of an authority figure imposing a sanction, positive or negative, on a subordinate. It is not the action of a peer imposing a sanction, positive or negative, on a colleague. Accountability, as a word, according to Bailey (1998), does not exist. Account on the other hand has several definitions, including "to be responsible to answer: with for" (1998). Accountability then is not something someone else can impose upon us. It is something we must do for ourselves by accepting responsibility and answering to those we serve with or for our actions (1998).

Gatekeepers hold themselves and their behaviors, actions, and practice accountable to those they serve. Simply, accountable behavior instills trust (Covey and Merrill, 2006). If gatekeepers are not more accountable, than responsibility to own who they are, has not been accepted. In turn, others will not trust us as respected partners in health care. Gatekeepers will only be engaged to the level of perceived accountability for practice with others. If that is only as a member of a health care team to carry out delegated practice, then we have created an image that is not reflective of the ability and responsibility of the nurse and nursing profession. Sadly, this is very descriptive of many of the nursing care settings today.

Accountability Communicates our Integrity and Professional Responsibility

Becoming accountable as a gatekeeper in health care requires that the gatekeeper not only accept responsibility but practice with integrity. Gatekeepers must be willing to evaluate their work honestly and determine if they are practicing according to the professional scopes and standards of nursing practice. If that practice is outside of the professional scopes and standards of nursing practice the gatekeeper must realign his or her practice.

How does the gatekeeper become accountable?

How is practice aligned professionally?

First one must clearly understand the professional scopes and standards for nursing practice. These can be obtained through the American Nurses Association or online through a web search. Understanding the boundaries of nursing practice and refusing to practice outside of these standards demonstrates accountability. The gatekeeper must accept responsibility and be accountable to educate others on these scopes and standards of nursing practice, role modeling for others verses falling victim to an erosion of the professional nursing image. Not understanding the role of the gatekeeper and the scopes and standards of nursing practice places the gatekeeper at risk for professional manipulation by non-nursing professionals. In this situation, the gatekeeper may be challenged to practice outside of the professional standard and often times may not know the difference.

Second, one should recognize that nursing is not a stand-alone profession. Gatekeepers are independent in practice, yet in health care we must collaborate. In this collaborative role gatekeepers must understand and be respectful of the professional scopes and standards of other professions without sacrificing their own.

Gatekeepers must be accountable "with for" (Baily, 1998) the patient they serve.

Third, the gatekeeper must be "politically" active. Gatekeepers must refuse to give control over their practice to anyone outside of the profession of nursing. Gatekeepers must accept responsibility and hold themselves accountable to write nursing care policy, to be active on service committees, to lead quality assurance, and refuse to fall victim within the environment they serve.

Accountability Can Change the Common Health Care Environment

To bring clarity to this discussion, I would like to share a personal experience. I was hired into a nursing management position at a time when the unit I was hired to manage and lead was in great turmoil. The unit was understaffed, Registered Nurse (RN) to patient ratios were often 1 nurse to 10 patients. Licensed Practical Nurses (LPN) assumed the care of 7 of the 10 patients with supposed oversight by the Registered Nurse. Nursing Assistants (NA) were utilized. However, they were shared between nurses and held ratios at times of up to 20 patients per nursing assistant.

Due to patient acuity RNs failed to properly oversee the LPN, leaving the LPN to practice outside of their scope and standard of nursing practice.

Incomplete physical care of patients occurred because the NA did not have clarity in their role as a result of being spread so thin and being responsible to more than one delegating RN who, in an overwhelmed state, could not delegate effectively. To create a vision, gate-keepers were running about trying to keep up, losing information, not gaining proper assessment, and not directing or controlling the flow of care because of significant work flow issues and no delivery of care structure.

Nursing task interventions such as the taking of vital signs, ambulation of patients, and patient teaching was not getting completed. In this situation, gatekeepers complained. Blame was placed on the organization for poor working conditions without recognition of the gatekeeper's role in the organization. Gatekeepers filed grievances with the union requesting mandates for safer working conditions.

The issue was that nurses did not own the role of the gatekeeper, failing to accept responsibility and maintain accountability for their professional service as a professional nurse. This led to an environment where non-nurse professionals controlled and dictated the care that was provided. By default, physicians accepted the responsibility and held themselves accountable to write orders for basic nursing care. These orders included tasks like taking vital signs every four hours in stable patients who would not require more than one time per day or shift. When meeting with these physicians to determine the need for this, the response received was that these orders were to assure that a gatekeeper or somebody will at least physically see their patients during a shift. What resulted in this unit was a mindset among physicians, administrators, and other health care professionals, even the gatekeepers themselves, that nursing care could not be performed without the direction of a physician.

As a gatekeeper, being accountable meant that I needed to help this team create change within this environment. It was as much my responsibility, as it was of every gatekeeper working in this unit, to assure that those we served received high quality care.

Creating change was not easy. It involved a significant amount of risk. It would have been very easy to hide within a soft image of caring, allowing non-nurse professionals to continue to lead and direct nursing care. Instead, I opened myself and our team up to collaborative partnerships, identified and utilized resources, educated each gatekeeper and non-nurse professional on the scopes and standards of professional nursing practice, and successfully implemented and maintained a Relationship Based Care Nursing Model.

Through the role modeling of my own accountability gatekeepers were empowered and began to develop their independent and collaborative roles within the health care team. Each gatekeeper began to take ownership for who he or she was as a nurse and began to blame less on those around them. As a result, patient care and quality improved creating an environment of respect for the role of the gatekeeper and for their professional practice. Physicians began to trust and depend on nursing judgment in care. The relationships became a primary focus and respect for the partnership between nurse and physician, nurse and nurse, nurse and other health care professionals, and nurse and patient developed. As the gatekeeper began to accept their own responsibility and hold themselves accountable to practice within the boundaries of their scopes and standards of professional practice, we saw an increase in satisfaction, quality, financial stability, and nurse led care. The gatekeepers in this unit grew in their own image of what nursing truly is and held themselves accountable, becoming strong advocates for their professional roles and responsibilities.

In ending this chapter, I leave you with a challenge.

Understand that as a nurse our profession is only governed by nurses. We have the *responsibility* to be *accountable* and to practice nursing with full authority within our independent as well as collaborative and delegated roles according to our scopes and standards of professional practice. As nurses, we have the obligation to *own* who we are, to serve as *gatekeepers*, with the authority to advocate, change health care environments, delegate, develop and implement policy, design and direct delivery of care, communicate and role model our professional duty, upholding the highest standard in quality and service to others.

Chapter Three Self-Reflection Challenges

Reflect on a time as a gatekeeper that you were challenged to provide care outside of the boundaries of your scopes and standards of nursing practice.

_____

_____

_____

_____

_____

_____

_____

_____

_____

_____

_____

_____

_____

_____

_____

_____

_____

_____

Describe how this made you feel.

_____

_____

_____

_____

_____

_____

_____

_____

_____

_____

_____

_____

_____

_____

_____

_____

_____

_____

_____

_____

Did you accept responsibility and hold yourself accountable to not practice outside of your professional boundaries? If yes, how? If no, why not?

_____

_____

_____

_____

_____

_____

_____

_____

_____

_____

_____

_____

_____

_____

_____

_____

What can you do for yourself professionally that will help you maintain accountability as a gatekeeper in health care?

_____

_____

_____

_____

_____

_____

_____

_____

_____

_____

_____

_____

_____

_____

_____

_____

_____

_____

Gatekeepers Embrace Power

As gatekeepers, we must embrace power. Power is neither good nor bad. Rather, "having power gives one the potential to change the attitudes and behaviors of individual people or groups" (Marquis & Huston, 2012). Considering the current attitudes and behaviors of nurses today, keeping this definition in mind is very important.

The nursing profession today remains primarily a female profession. Throughout history, women have been socialized to think differently about power, and in many cases assign a negative connotation to the use or application of this power (2012). This is not an excuse for the ongoing co-dependent nature of thinking within the nursing profession, or the negative thinking toward power that surrounds the position of the gatekeeper. It is important, however to acknowledge that gender has influenced the self-image of the gatekeeper and, as a result, the nursing profession. This has promoted a reluctance to take ownership for the full role of the gatekeeper.

Unfortunately, this means that although nursing education has progressed and we declare ourselves an independent profession gatekeepers collectively, as a professional body, have not effectively embraced the power necessary within leadership roles both formal and informal to eliminate the barriers that threaten professional independence in nursing (2012).

Understanding the Barrier to Power Acceptance

The barriers that threaten the power of the gatekeeper are self-perpetuated. To eliminate them, gatekeepers must recognize the behaviors that demonstrate a promotion of a weak and negative image. Gatekeepers must accept the responsibility to change these behaviors to promote the independent and collaborative authority of the professional nurse.

There are many ways to embrace power. One of the greatest and most powerful ways is through a willingness to communicate accomplishments. When gatekeepers fail to demonstrate who they are and what they do as a nursing professional there is a failure in communicating to others the powerful image and full authority of the professional nurse and the nursing profession.

It is important for gatekeepers to communicate through many forums the image of the nurse. Gatekeepers manage and coordinate the care of others. Gatekeepers heal. Gatekeepers protect. Gatekeepers discover. Gatekeepers cure, and much more. Power is established by a willingness to accept responsibility, be accountable, and own who we are.

As gatekeepers, nurses are surrounded by many colleagues who are brave, willing to take risks, and accept responsibility and accountability for their professional role. These gatekeepers are excellent role models and spark desire in others to practice with the same convictions and demonstration of their powerful role. These gatekeepers are listened to and respected. Their opinions and recommendations on the care of others matter.

As gatekeepers, however, nurses are also surrounded by colleagues who are not in control, who complain, are disorganized, and may be passive, passive aggressive, or even abusive in nature. With this image the gatekeeper forfeits power. This gatekeeper becomes powerless. This professional nurse is not respected but rather feared or ignored by others. As a professional that speaks and role models from a position of powerlessness the gatekeeper will never gain the respect individually or collaboratively in representation of the nursing profession as a partner in the management of care.

Understanding What It Takes

Gatekeepers must begin to understand that it takes each individual professional nurse to practice from a place of power to create a positive image and demonstrate a powerful profession. Reflect on this for a moment. Think about your role as a gatekeeper.

What behaviors do you communicate to others?

Do they represent a position of power or powerlessness?

I am now going to make a very bold statement. If you are a gatekeeper who communicates and represents the profession from a powerless position, get out of the profession or change your behavior. Hurting the image of the nursing profession does not demonstrate a willingness to do what is right for those we serve. The squeaky wheel may get the grease. However, it does not get respect. Powerful and safe patient care is established when gatekeepers take ownership for their professional role, accept responsibility to practice as a professional, hold themselves personally and professionally accountable, and demonstrate respect for others as well as themselves.

Demonstrating a Powerful Image Can Be Simple

To demonstrate a powerful moment in nursing I would like to share a personal experience. Several years ago, when in my nursing management position, I was rounding with patients and staff in my unit. As I rounded a corner, I spotted a gatekeeper doing a dance in the hallway. Others were laughing and clapping their hands. It was a very happy moment, as well as a powerful one, for in that moment I could see the pride these gatekeepers felt for the role they played in patient care.

When I asked why this gatekeeper was dancing, she quickly responded "because we just gave a very successful enema! It took several of us but the patient is happy and we are happy!"

Not long after this public celebration of success, I received a phone call from the Chief Executive Officer (CEO) of this organization. He communicated that he was calling because he received a complaint and wanted to know what to do about it. The complaint received was received from gatekeepers in another unit. These gatekeepers took offense to the laughter and happiness of the nurses in our unit.

Before I could respond, both of us began to laugh. We agreed nothing should be done. Case closed. A gatekeeper should celebrate success and assure that all hear of that success. The power of this moment influenced another department! Others in the organization began to ask why they were not celebrating and rejoicing in their work. Slowly things began to change.

A successful enema is small compared to the many successes of gatekeepers today. Gatekeepers everywhere are starting businesses, leading research, publishing, curing patients, caring, and more. Through the communication of accomplishments and the celebration of success, big or small, the profession of nursing and each individual and independent yet collaborative gatekeeper can "change the attitudes and behaviors" (Marquis & Huston, 2012) of others. Now, this is powerful stuff.

In ending of this chapter, I leave you with a challenge.

Understand that as nurses our profession is only governed by nurses. We have the *power*, and the *responsibility*, to be *accountable* and to practice nursing with full authority within our independent as well as collaborative and delegated roles according to our scopes and standards of professional practice. As nurses, we have the obligation to *own* who we are, to serve as *gatekeepers*, with the authority to advocate, change health care environments, delegate, develop and implement policy, design and direct delivery of care, communicate, and role model our professional duty, upholding the highest standard in quality and service to others.

Chapter Four Self-Reflection Challenges

Reflect on your response earlier in this chapter. Do you represent the profession of nursing and serve as a gatekeeper from a position of power? If yes, how? If no, why not?

_____

_____

_____

_____

_____

_____

_____

_____

_____

_____

_____

_____

_____

_____

_____

_____

_____

What can you do to strengthen your position of power or to change your behavior to reflect a position of power as a gatekeeper in health care?

_____

_____

_____

_____

_____

_____

_____

_____

_____

_____

_____

_____

_____

_____

_____

_____

_____

_____

Why is it important for our patients, colleagues, collaborative partners and the nursing profession that as a gatekeeper you practice from a position of power?

_____

_____

_____

_____

_____

_____

_____

_____

_____

_____

_____

_____

_____

_____

_____

_____

Gatekeepers Empower Others

As gatekeepers, we both empower ourselves and others. This means that as professional nurses gatekeepers take attention off of themselves and work to help other gatekeepers own who they are, accept responsibility for their role, and maintain accountability in their practice.

Gatekeeper's role model endlessly, understanding that it is their responsibility to assure that the profession of nursing remains strong in the care of others. Figuratively speaking, great gatekeepers work themselves out of a job by empowering those they serve. Only through this level of empowerment will a gatekeeper gain the power and respect to secure his or her position.

Practicing to Our Full Potential Is a Necessity

As gatekeepers, assuring that we practice to our full potential is a necessity in today's health care climate. Kunic and Jackson (2013) identify the key message from the Institute of Medicine Report to be that "all nurses should practice to the full extent of their education and training". They also argue that it is time to remove the barriers that prevent nurses from reaching their full potential in practice (2013).

Developing potential and removing barriers is a responsibility that belongs to the gatekeeper. Historically, our co-dependent culture has promoted an attitude of powerless-ness. As a result we have fallen victim to this culture and have created barriers that prevent us from empowering each other to develop as powerful, individual and collaborative gate-keepers. These barriers include but are not limited to a failure to own who we are in our image, practicing from a passive role as an advocate in the avoidance of conflict and challenge, a lack of support and encouragement for the success and advancement of each other, and a lack of understanding of our full responsibility in the management of the care of others in relation to our professional scopes and standards of practice.

A failure to empower each other and accept the responsibility to eliminate these barriers results in a profession that looks to and relies on others to make decisions and provide direction for our practice. Responsibility is displaced, accountability is lacking, and power is given away. This provides opportunity for others to decide the worth of nursing and the nursing profession. If gatekeepers are to reach their full potential in practice they must understand and embrace their authority to empower themselves and others by gaining control over the roles and responsibilities of the professional nurse.

Achieving Empowerment

Gatekeepers empower themselves and others by sharing knowledge and developing a sense of competence (MacPhee, Skelton-Green, Gouthillette & Suryaprakash, 2011). For example, through the art of delegation the gatekeeper teaches and role models skills and behaviors, empowering others to learn and grow. This strengthens the level of quality in the care being provided.

Gatekeepers have a responsibility to train other gatekeepers, facilitating and directing their learning. Gatekeepers have the responsibility to be lifelong learners to assure they have the ability to empower others. Through gaining and sharing knowledge and positive support and guidance of others the gatekeeper will be empowered and others will as well.

Embracing our Professional Collective Responsibility

Through empowerment, gatekeepers embrace the profession and demonstrate support for one another. Differences are accepted and the profession benefits from the practice of independent and collaborative nursing professionals that have different backgrounds, values, and belief systems. Even with this individuality, it can be discovered that gatekeepers share a common background, set of values, and beliefs in nursing that make us one.

Gatekeepers serve in many roles and have many responsibilities. In those roles and responsibilities insight is gained from other professionals and gatekeepers are afforded the opportunity to develop different skill sets. It is important to understand, however, that there is only one set of defined scopes and standards of practice for nursing professionals and only one code of ethics. Nurses therefore, govern nurses. In order to empower themselves and others within the profession there must be a relationship between gatekeepers such as a mentorship or preceptorship that allows for insightful exchange of assessment and evaluation of the gatekeepers' strengths and weaknesses.

Speaking and practicing as a gatekeeper from one professional voice is powerful. In this empowered state, gatekeepers demonstrate a commitment to advancing nursing practice, advancing nursing education, and assuring the profession of nursing leads health care in demonstrating that only the highest quality and standard of care be delivered to those we serve.

Reflection on Empowerment

One of the earliest and most empowering moments in my career was the time I spent in nursing school. The Dean of our Nursing Program understood the value in taking the time to empower others. I was given the opportunity to attend meetings, and travel and join her on a State Advisory Board, developing my skills in nursing leadership. This experience afforded to me by another gatekeeper ignited energy and a passion to focus my professional commitment on improving outcomes in nursing and health care organizations and making a difference in the quality and service to others.

I admired this gatekeeper then and still today. She did not serve the nursing profession and those she cared for from a place of fear for her own position. She served with a realization that by empowering others her own position would be stronger, she would be respected, and most importantly, the profession of nursing would advance and those we cared for would benefit from our strength as leaders and gatekeepers of care.

Many nurses can tell a horror story of the nurse that belittled them during training. Many of us can recall our feelings of powerlessness in this experience and the increase in our anxiety as a result. In life, and within our profession, the negative experiences often remain at the forefront of our actions and behaviors and over time can shape the way we practice, regardless of our desire to not let that happen. Just like the Dean in my story, we must resist this negativity and individually role model our empowered state to create generations of empowered gatekeepers, through ongoing positive support for each other.

In ending this chapter, I leave you with a challenge.

Understand that as nurses our profession is only governed by nurses. We have the *power*, and the *responsibility* to be *accountable* and to practice nursing with full authority within our independent as well as collaborative and delegated roles according to our scopes and standards of professional practice. As nurses, we have the obligation to *own* who we are, to *empower* ourselves and others, to serve as *gatekeepers,* with the authority to advocate, change health care environments, delegate, develop and implement policy, design and direct delivery of care, communicate, and role model our professional duty, upholding the highest standard in quality and service to others.

Chapter Five Self-Reflection Challenges

List the activities you participate in that empower you as a gatekeeper and describe what you have learned from them.

_____

_____

_____

_____

_____

_____

_____

_____

_____

_____

_____

_____

_____

_____

_____

_____

_____

_____

_____

List the names of other gatekeepers you have mentored or taught as a preceptor in the last year.

_____

_____

_____

_____

_____

_____

_____

_____

_____

_____

_____

_____

_____

_____

_____

_____

_____

What learning from your self-empowerment opportunities did you share with those gatekeepers?

_____

_____

_____

_____

_____

_____

_____

_____

_____

_____

_____

_____

_____

_____

_____

_____

What more can you do in your nursing practice to role model empowerment and to empower others through your service?

_____

_____

_____

_____

_____

_____

_____

_____

_____

_____

_____

_____

_____

_____

_____

_____

Are you willing to seek out a mentor and to serve as a mentor for another? Why? Why not?

_____

_____

_____

_____

_____

_____

_____

_____

_____

_____

_____

_____

_____

_____

_____

_____

_____

_____

Gatekeepers Practice with Courage

As gatekeepers, we must practice with courage. Courage is a virtue we are expected to have and somehow from the moment we begin our journey to becoming a nurse we are supposed to develop the courage to uphold the standards of practice for nursing without waiver. Gatekeepers must practice and uphold these standards in the face of conflict, through ethical and moral challenges, and when others fail to do so themselves. This virtue lends to an image that the gatekeeper must be strong and a reality that in order to be strong gatekeepers must maintain a position of power and demonstrate ownership for the nursing professionals they are.

Courage is not a virtue that calls for silence. The idea that gatekeepers silently suffer assuming the burdens of those they care for is a misguided image. Gatekeepers at all levels must find their voice. Gatekeepers must have the courage to express their knowledge about nursing practice, about physiological and psychological systems, about the purpose and effect of medication, about actual and foreseen outcomes of care, and so much more.

Courage means that as a gatekeeper we practice with integrity, honesty, and foreseeability. It means that we role model not just the "soft stuff" but the things that keep our patients safe in our care. Having courage means that, as gatekeepers, we own our responsibility and do our part to empower other gatekeepers to practice according to the professional nursing scopes and standards of practice. Having courage means that, as gatekeepers, we uphold our professional code of ethics. Having courage means that, as gatekeepers, we do not allow fear to delay or curtail our responses, that we learn to trust our intuition and respond appropriately, and to face another health partner with an opposing view.

A Demonstration of Courage

Courage is more than an expression. It is demonstrated in action. While working as a staff nurse in a medical surgical unit, I cared for an elderly patient suffering from cardiac and respiratory issues who at the time was very frail. This patient was placed on a nothing, by, mouth diet and had not eaten in over 48 hours. There was an intravenous solution infusing to keep her hydrated and offer electrolytes. However, to paint a clear picture this patient suffered from muscle wasting and a declining loss of function.

During my shift, I received a call from this patient's physician, who I respect professionally. This physician gave me an order in response to lab values reported earlier in the day. The order was to administer an IV medication STAT. I did take the order. However, not being familiar with the drug, I held myself accountable to research it and discuss it with the pharmacist prior to administration. It was discovered that this drug has a warning associated with it. The warning was that even in IV form it should not be administered to a person with an empty stomach. If not administered with food it could cause gastrointestinal bleeding.

Without question, I contacted the physician and shared this. The physician became very upset and demanded that the medication be administered. The physician accused me of stepping outside of my boundaries in questioning the safety of this order and told me to focus on my role in carrying out the order. Well, as you can imagine or may be feeling in response to this, it took me by surprise as well as infuriated me that this physician knew so little about and demonstrated little respect for our professional responsibilities as gatekeepers in care.

At that moment, however, I could not spend time arguing or educating this physician as there was a patient involved who needed care. I needed to find my courage to do what was right. It would have been very easy to avoid further conflict and administer this drug. If something went wrong, I could have just stated in the court of law that the physician told me to do it, right? Wrong!

I repeated the risk again and informed the physician that out of a duty for the safety of my patient and in alignment with my scopes and standards of practice I could not administer this drug without feeding the patient as well. Again, the physician did not take kindly and accused me of telling her how to do her job. I then communicated with courage, strength, and conviction that due to the safety risks of this medication she would need to administer the medication herself if it needed to be adminis- tered without food.

Now, as you can imagine an angry physician can make life difficult. In this case my direct manager was notified of my refusal to administer this medication. My courage led to the risk of receiving a disciplinary action or, even worse, a termination for refusal of care. I held my ground, however, because I know it was right and I had my scopes and standards of nursing practice and my code of ethics on hand. In review, my nurse manager supported my decision.

The physician, however, did choose to administer this medication. I assured I had documented my decision not to support this, and used my courage to remain at the side of this patient while the physician performed the administration of medication. This was not easy. However, I will never regret this decision. Shortly after administration, the patient began to bleed. Setting differences aside as professionals the physician and I worked together to stabilize the patient and no serious outcomes occurred. Without further words to each other, we went on our way to care for the rest of our patients that day.

Now, I would like to share why having this courage was so important beyond the safety of this patient's care. At the end of this physician's day, I received a phone call. In the hours that has separated us this physician took time to reflect on and understand the boundaries of a gatekeeper's professional licensure and the responsibility a gatekeeper has to challenge a decision as an advocate for safety. This physician then displayed her own courage as a professional to call me and apologize for such condescending behavior and disregard for working together as independent and collaborative professionals. In that moment each of us gained respect for the other.

This example is just one of many of the experiences of gatekeepers at all levels. The message is simple. As a gatekeeper you have accepted the calling, and responsibility, to hold another human life in your hands, to keep safe, to protect, to heal, care, and cure! Think of the power this has. Own it, accept the responsibility, and be accountable as a gatekeeper to use your courage to always do what is right.

In ending this chapter, I leave you with a challenge.

Understand that as nurses our profession is only governed by nurses. We have the *power*, and the *responsibility* to be *accountable* and to practice nursing with *courage* and full authority within our independent as well as collaborative and delegated roles according to our scopes and standards of professional practice. As nurses, we have the obligation to *own* who we are, to serve as *gatekeepers*, with the authority to advocate, change health care environments, delegate, develop and implement policy, design and direct delivery of care, communicate, and role model our professional duty, upholding the highest standard in quality and service to others.

Chapter Six Self-Reflection Challenges

Describe a situation when you had to use your courage.

_____

_____

_____

_____

_____

_____

_____

_____

_____

_____

_____

_____

_____

_____

_____

_____

_____

_____

Describe a situation when you failed to use your courage or you wished you had used more courage.

_____

_____

_____

_____

_____

_____

_____

_____

_____

_____

_____

_____

_____

_____

_____

_____

_____

_____

_____

_____

On a scale of 1-10, with 1 being the least and 10 being the most, rate your level of courage in professional practice. Reflect on why you rated yourself as you did.

_____

_____

_____

_____

_____

_____

_____

_____

_____

_____

_____

_____

_____

_____

_____

_____

_____

_____

_____

What can you do in your professional practice to improve your level of courage?

_____

_____

_____

_____

_____

_____

_____

_____

_____

_____

_____

_____

_____

_____

_____

_____

_____

What can you do in your professional practice to help other gatekeepers develop their courage?

_____

_____

_____

_____

_____

_____

_____

_____

_____

_____

_____

_____

_____

_____

_____

_____

_____

_____

Gatekeepers are Political

As gatekeepers, we must engage politically. It is necessary for nurses to learn how to navigate a formal organizational system effectively. Just like power, being political is neither good nor bad. It is just a necessary responsibility to ensure the progression of the nursing profession and for the benefit of those we serve.

Relationships Are Key

Politics occurs at every level of nursing and the most effective gatekeeper in regards to maneuvering through a political arena is the one who focuses on building and maintaining positive relationships in the environment of care. Although the term politics was used explicitly in Manion's book *Management and Leadership, Practical Strategies for Health Care Leaders* (2005), she discusses "The Art of Effectively Facilitating Processes."

To do this, gatekeepers must be active in their work. They must be trustworthy and practice with integrity. A gatekeeper must build positive relationships to assure a level of influence that actively affects all care processes in a positive way. In building relationships, gatekeepers do not have to strive to make all people happy or ensure that they are liked by everyone. I mean that as gatekeepers you practice from a foundation of evidence that supports your practice. It means that you have gained respect as a gatekeeper for owning who you are, accepting responsibility, and practicing with accountability, courage, and power.

It is important to recognize that, generally, we cannot make others happy and we cannot make everyone like us. True happiness comes from within. If someone does not have it, it is not your fault. Blaming others for a lack of happiness weakens political power and causes people to practice from a place of powerlessness. Worrying about being liked verses respected distracts us from our purpose of serving others and will misguide us along the path to safe patient care. Being political means that others are persuaded to believe in your message. It is about getting things done for those we serve as for our own professional growth.

Action Speaks Louder than Words

Engaging in the work environment is just the beginning of the political process for a gatekeeper. To be effective in the facilitation of processes (Manion, 2010), a gatekeeper must be active. When a gatekeeper is active a gatekeeper becomes visible to others.

There are many ways for a gatekeeper to become active, visible, and participate in political action. Becoming a member of a professional nursing organization, participating in committee work within the organization, being active in shared governance processes, publishing activities, committing to lifelong learning and sharing that learning, and getting elected to a formal seat in your city, state, or federal government are just a few.

However, a gatekeeper can be political simply by taking responsibility and being accountable to communicate and role model a professional image of nursing.

For a gatekeeper, "it never hurts to toot your own horn once in a while" (Blanchard, Lacinak, Tompkins, and Ballard, 2002).

The Impact of Political Discomfort

From time to time, nursing students will ask why being political is necessary in the nursing profession. This question comes from a place of discomfort and lack of know how. It is understandable, that some will be uncomfortable with this responsibility. Gatekeepers need to understand that choosing to remain comfortable, however, allows others to create an image of the professional nurse that is not accurate and this image weakens the power base of the profession as whole.

The profession of nursing is made up of individual gatekeepers or nurses. If nursing is truly an independent and collaborative profession, as stated by Florence Nightingale (Selandres & Patrick, 2012) then each individual gatekeeper should be actively doing what is right for those we serve. If each gatekeeper chooses to be politically passive, standardization verses individualization of care will continue under direction of those outside of the profession.

Gatekeepers are viewed by our communities as caring professionals. However, caring does not only mean communicating an image of a guardian angel, caring hands, or the lady with the lamp. Caring means gatekeepers use their voice and take charge and ownership of the professional responsibility to be active in the care of others. Through political action gatekeepers serve as advocates, change agents, and visionaries for high quality care.

Advancing Practice through Political Action

In chapter 3, I presented a personal experience of assisting a team in chaos as a nurse manager. The gatekeepers in this example were looking for others to solve their problems and lacked engagement for their professional responsibility within the organization. Politically they were not visible. They did not use their voice or their action to navigate within the organization. This type of activity was not something they perceived as a part of their job and it resulted in high nurse to patient ratios, poor quality outcomes, and a lack of trust in their ability to perform safe patient care without physician and administrative direction.

My role as a gatekeeper and manager was to help these nurses realize their responsibility for political action in order to make change and improve outcomes. To do this, I role modeled the importance of collaboration with other nursing colleagues and health care professionals.

We demonstrated that networking and communication was important to develop an understanding of the issues surrounding nursing practice in this unit. It became clear that making change and being politically active involves the influence and engagement of more than one person and is a necessary component in building positive relationships to "facilitate processes" (Manion, 2010).

These gatekeepers were encouraged to participate in unit committees, and group sessions to discuss the barriers surrounding nursing practice and delivery of care in this unit. Through this engagement change was facilitated and nurses were empowered to take action. It was necessary to allow these gate-keepers to express their values as independent and collaborative professionals in nursing. Each gatekeeper needed to have the opportunity through this political activity to realize that collectively they shared many of the same values and vision for what the practice of nursing should be.

Through this experience gatekeepers were educated and realigned with their responsibility and authority to practice according to the scopes and standards of practice for nursing and the code of ethics. From this, awareness was achieved and these gatekeepers began to take ownership for this professional responsibility, they were empowered, and engaging in political activity throughout the organization for the benefit of nursing and patient care outcomes.

This was an amazing transformation that took place. Physicians and other health care professionals began to trust in each individual gatekeeper. As a result, admission referrals, physician, staff, and patient satisfaction increased, nursing satisfaction increased, registered nurse turnover decreased, and union grievances decreased. Every gatekeeper began to feel empowered and they began to empower each other to take control over the management of patient care in that environment.

For the standards of nursing practice and the image of independent and collaborative practice to be known, it must be the gatekeeper that communicates through political activity and it must be the gatekeeper that role models the message. It must be consistent. Gatekeepers must be willing to serve, to broaden their shoulders, and to work well with others. The gatekeeper should have a presence in any organization not because the organization supports it but because the gatekeeper demonstrates the expectation. This presence should be so strong and visible that respect for our professional knowledge and experience is given. They should own it and communicate it! Gatekeepers are the only ones that can.

In ending this chapter, I leave you with this, our growing challenge.

Understand that as nurses our profession is only governed by nurses. We have the *power*, and the *responsibility* to be *accountable*, *political* and to practice nursing with *courage* and full authority within our independent as well as collaborative and delegated roles according to our scopes and standards of professional practice. Nurses, we have the obligation to *own* who we are, to serve as *gatekeepers*, with the authority to advocate, change health care environments, delegate, develop and implement policy, design and direct delivery of care, communicate, and role model our professional duty, upholding the highest standard in quality and service to others.

Chapter Seven Self-Reflection Challenges

Why is being politically active such an important responsibility for the gatekeeper to accept?

_____

_____

_____

_____

_____

_____

_____

_____

_____

_____

_____

_____

_____

_____

_____

_____

_____

_____

In what ways have you as a gatekeeper engaged in political activity in your organization and in the profession of nursing?

_____

_____

_____

_____

_____

_____

_____

_____

_____

_____

_____

_____

_____

_____

_____

_____

_____

What can you do to become more politically active as a gatekeeper in your organization and in health care?

_____

_____

_____

_____

_____

_____

_____

_____

_____

_____

_____

_____

_____

_____

_____

_____

_____

_____

How can you empower other gatekeepers to become politically engaged in or outside o f the work environment?

_____

_____

_____

_____

_____

_____

_____

_____

_____

_____

_____

_____

_____

_____

_____

_____

_____

_____

Gatekeepers Realize Their Spiritual Presence

As gatekeepers we realize our spiritual presence and practice with an awareness of our spiritual presence. It must be understood that spirituality is not a religion. It is a sense of being, of inner connectivity with something greater than ourselves. Some say it is a guiding energy.

In Our Image We Are Spiritual

Related to nursing care, spirituality is a guiding internal force that leads the gatekeeper to knowledge and understanding. Whether all gatekeepers recognize themselves as spiritual people or not, it is important to understand that those we serve do. In this spiritual presence others gain a sense of trust, comfort, and security in the care the gatekeeper provides.

Because of this presence, some will blindly follow the direction of the gatekeeper. It is important that the trust others have in us is not broken by a failure to connect with our inner self, by recognizing that feeling within us that alerts us when something is not right, causing a failure to practice and serve according to our standards of practice and code of ethics.

It is wrong to alter the positive feelings of comfort and security others have in the healing hands of the gatekeeper by denying this spiritual presence and closing ourselves off to the inner feelings that lead us to do the right thing for every person in our care, for ourselves, and our profession.

Connecting Through Self-Awareness

For some, spirituality is a sensitive subject. I believe this is due to differences in opinion about what spirituality is. Spirituality is often thought of as something private. In our calling to care, however, gatekeepers must learn to be open to their spirituality by developing a strong sense of self-awareness. This self-awareness allows for a connection with the inner-self that prompts the gatekeeper to use courage, to be responsible, to be accountable, to be powerful, and so much more.

How do gatekeepers gain this self-awareness or learn how to open themselves up to their spiritual being?

They do so, simply, by listening and allowing the feelings that occur in response to every situation to speak to them. These feelings, for example may be experienced as calm, anxiety, heaviness, or worry. We often identify this as intuition or a sense of knowing. It is important to recognize and validate these feelings through quiet reflection and review.

In his book on *Radical Loving Care, Building the Healing Hospital In America* (2005), Erie Chapman discussed the need for gatekeepers to learn to focus on the "loving side of us" (page 93). In application to nursing practice, this "loving side of us" involves an understanding that the gatekeeper has a spiritual presence. Chapman also notes that the noise of our everyday activity interrupts our connection with this presence, keeping us so busy that we do not take the time to pay attention to what matters most (page 93).

In consideration of our professional responsibilities as gatekeepers in health care, nurses are often focused on and overwhelmed with the day-to-day tasks, missing the point of their purpose. This results in a failure to role model our true value as independent and collaborative practitioners in health care. Gatekeepers short change themselves, their patients, their colleagues and others by setting aside their spiritual attention in their busy day and failing to recognize the power they have with each human to human encounter.

It is the responsibility of each and every gatekeeper, in an effort to take ownership for who they are as a nurse, to slow down, listen to their inner-self, connect to their spiritual being, re-train their mindset, and understand the value of the gatekeeper is not to get caught up in the tasks that are performed but rather the action surrounding those tasks to assure we maintain the trust, comfort, and security of those we serve.

Believing the Message

Whether every gatekeeper believes in this message or not, it is a matter for consideration. Historically, the spiritual image has been created for us. Think back to the beginning of this book and to the discussion about the image of the nurse that is created by those we serve. Gatekeepers are thought of as guardian angels, a set of caring hands, a mirror image of Florence Nightingale, the lady with the lamp. Gatekeepers keep watch and protect those in need. For this reason, it is the responsibility of the gatekeeper to communicate and role model this spiritual image as not only a soft one but something powerful. It is important to bring meaning to what true caring is and to be accountable to those we serve by keeping ourselves open to the inner-self and to develop our spiritual connection in relation to the care of others.

The Connection that Saved a Life

As I recall a personal situation that demonstrates how the spiritual connection of the gatekeeper works, I ask you:

How many times have you as a gatekeeper experienced an inner gut feeling that something was not right with your patient?

Have you ever questioned where this feeling comes from?

Have you ever made reference or heard others make reference to this feeling as a "divine intervention?"

In my own experience as a gatekeeper, I have. I recall entering a patient's room one night just to say hello. The patient was in good spirits, was talkative, and looked comfortable. Something, however, did not feel right. Instantly my inner-self spoke to me through a feeling of something heavy and anxious in my gut. I needed to take action, but did not know why.

Although the patient looked and acted just fine, I listened to this gut feeling and responded. I contacted the physician, I provided him with a report noting stable vital signs and assessment but expressing my feelings of concern. Once he heard my report, he expressed concern over my lack of judgment in making this phone call. As you can imagine, I am sure he was thinking that I was not very skilled. To call a physician on a gut feeling of impending doom was not scientific. Receiving no orders to work collaboratively with the physician at that time, I accepted the responsibility, in response to my intuitive feeling, to independently practice as a professional nurse within my scopes and standards of professional practice.

I monitored this patient closely, even placing a heart monitor on him to observe his cardiac status. Within one hour of contacting the physician, this patient began to bleed, and bleed profusely, both orally and rectally. His blood pressure plummeted and he required an immediate transfer to the intensive care unit. I believe we saved this patient's life on that day because of a divine intervention. My care very quickly transitioned from one of independence to one of complete collaboration. This patient received an overwhelming number of units of packed red blood cells over the course of a couple of days, I recall somewhere around 21, and the bleeding did stop. I think back to that moment now and get chills. If I did not realize my spiritual presence and ignored or dismissed my inner-self this patient may not have lived.

In ending this chapter, I leave you with our challenge.

Understand that as nurses our profession is only governed by nurses. We have the *power*, and the *responsibility* to be *accountable, political* and to practice nursing with *courage* and full authority within our independent as well as collaborative and delegated roles according to our scopes and standards of professional practice. As nurses, we have the obligation to *own* who we are, realize our *spiritual presence*, to serve as *gatekeepers*, with the authority to advocate, change health care environments, delegate, develop and implement policy, design and direct delivery of care, communicate, and role model our professional duty, upholding the highest standard in quality and service to others.

Chapter Eight Self-Reflection Challenges

Describe a situation when, as a gatekeeper, you failed to listen to your inner-self in the care of a patient. What was the outcome?

_____

_____

_____

_____

_____

_____

_____

_____

_____

_____

_____

_____

_____

_____

_____

_____

_____

_____

_____

_____

Reflecting upon the above situation, what do you believe prevented you from connecting to your inner-self in that moment?

_____

_____

_____

_____

_____

_____

_____

_____

_____

_____

_____

_____

_____

_____

_____

_____

_____

_____

Describe a scenario when you did listen to your inner-self in the care of a patient. What was the outcome?

_____

_____

_____

_____

_____

_____

_____

_____

_____

_____

_____

_____

_____

_____

_____

_____

_____

_____

_____

In both of these experiences, what have you learned in regards to the importance of developing a spiritual connection within yourself?

_____

_____

_____

_____

_____

_____

_____

_____

_____

_____

_____

_____

_____

_____

_____

_____

_____

In what ways can you develop the spiritual connection within yourself? Develop or outline a plan to develop this connection.

_____

_____

_____

_____

_____

_____

_____

_____

_____

_____

_____

_____

_____

_____

_____

_____

_____

_____

Gatekeepers Lead from All Levels

As gatekeepers we understand the responsibility for leadership and we lead from all levels. An ongoing argument in regard to leadership exists in whether leaders are born or taught. Most of us can argue both sides of this discussion and have it make sense. Ultimately, however, it does not matter. The argument in and of itself provides an avenue for gatekeepers to fail to take ownership of their responsibility to lead regardless of their position.

What does matter is that true leadership takes a conscious effort to do what is right. True leadership is not one of position. True leadership is role modeled and supportive of the greater profession. True leadership is powerful but only through the empowerment of others. Tomey, (2009), states that nursing leaders are knowledgeable, they are advocates, and they take risks, guided by philosophy in practice. This identifies each and every gatekeeper as a leader in practice today.

Taking Risk for the Benefit of Those We Serve

Learning to take risk is of great importance to our profession. All gatekeepers must accept the responsibility and hold themselves accountable to take personal risk for the benefit of those we serve. As gatekeepers, playing it safe will not advance the nursing profession. I am not advocating that we base our nursing practice on risk taking behaviors. I am, however, advocating that we must take risk to address those that are not practicing to a professional standard. We must have courage to stand up for what is right in the treatment of others. We must challenge ourselves to always do better and never settle for the status quo.

Most gatekeepers enter into nursing because they want to care for others. Many do this without fully understanding what the concept of caring really means. Caring means that we manage care and that we lead from all levels tirelessly, creating vision, empowering others, and transforming health care. It means that whether we have a quiet approach or a loud one, we always take the risk to do what is right. The patients and communities we serve depend on the strength of each and every gatekeeper. Vestal, (2010), recommends that to build this ability nurses must do something every day that scares us or forces us to come out of our comfort zone.

What have you done today, for the benefit of those we serve that scares you or forces you out of your comfort zone (2010)?

A Vision of Leadership

Again, leadership does not have to equate with a formal position. True leaders do not need the permission of a title or position to lead. If all gatekeepers accepted this responsibility, this book and the self-analysis it encourages would be unnecessary. All gatekeepers would own who they are, take responsibility, hold themselves accountable, embrace power, empower others, be political, practice with courage, and recognize their spiritual presence.

Whether you are an experienced gatekeeper or novice gatekeeper, reflect on your practice. There is no doubt that you have taken great risk from time to time in your career or on your journey to becoming a nurse. The questions that need to be asked are:

Do you role model this willingly and consistently in the care of others?

Do you empower other gatekeepers in their practice to do the same?

Do you contribute to nursing practice in your organization and in the greater professional community by actively participating on committees, such as, by assisting with the writing and management of nursing care policies and procedures?

Do you share your years of knowledge and experience, providing evidence of your value in practice?

Have you consistently allowed evidence based practice to guide your nursing care, and are you teaching others to do the same?

Are you respected as an independent and collaborative professional? If so, how? If not, Why?

Do you communicate a vision for excellence and work collaboratively with other gatekeepers to find commonality in this vision moving the profession forward in a supportive and positive way?

Take a moment to reflect on these questions and the answers you have provided.

A Message about Leadership

Regardless of your role in the nursing profession, do not be afraid to take risks. You should learn to walk the talk and role model your commitment to the profession and those you serve within your day to day behaviors (Jenkins & Stewart, 2010). Think back to the examples of positive and negative power or powerlessness earlier in this book. The professional image of every gatekeeper is needed to truly communicate who we are and what our role is in the greater community. Whether this is why you chose to be a gatekeeper or not it is your responsibility.

Gatekeepers must lead from all levels to build strength, demonstrate commitments, and remain strong as advocates for those we serve. Leading from all levels means that responsibility is shared regardless of the position you hold. I have heard novice nurses comment "what do I have to contribute. I don't have any experience." This is a disappointing statement and it brings about great frustration. The novice nurse has just as much to share in regards to new and better ways of doing things as an experienced nurse has to share what has worked and has not worked in practice over time.

Generational Tolerance Is Necessary for Leadership Development

As leaders in the profession of nursing it is necessary for every gatekeeper to demonstrate generational tolerance and accept the responsibility to promote leadership from all levels. Because of a generational intolerance, many gatekeepers do not perceive their role to include leadership. Novice nurses tend to forgo the responsibility as a response to learning their place in a working environment. Experienced nurses often complain that this is not in their job description, as they are hired to care for patients at the bedside. This may be the result of historical trends of co-dependency that have created a perpetual failure to lead, causing stress in the work place. Practice and literature have also utilized the term manager and leader interchangeably. This lends to confusion in practice that equates the leadership role with that of a nurse in a formal position. Often experienced nurses are those in those formal positions as a result of being an excellent practitioner verses a nurse with strong leadership skills.

As a gatekeeper it is important to resist the temptation to release the responsibility to lead to only those in formal positions. Years of practice experience does not equate to great leadership. It is imperative that as gatekeepers we utilize the nursing process to identify valuable skill sets in all colleagues regardless of their level of experience and practice and allow for the growth and development of leadership in each individual gatekeeper. Leadership is associated with a desire or commitment to serve (Jenkins & Stewart, 2010) and all gatekeepers regardless of the position they hold or experience they have, should have the desire and make the commitment to serve (2010).

Allowing for this growth can only strengthen our image. By encouraging others in our profession and taking the time to mentor and support we develop a strong base of leadership to lead our future. We have a responsibility to bridge the generations. By learning to be generationally tolerant, and supportive, leaders will develop at all levels. Through this development we assure a strong succession and gain power, establishing value as a respected profession in health care.

Always a Leader

Sharing a personal example in leadership, I will reflect on an earlier time in my career. I had been serving as a gatekeeper for about three years. I was working full time in a busy medical, surgical unit and when I arrived one morning for my shift I was informed that the delivery of care system had changed. Without preparation or warning each RN was responsible for a total of 12-16 patients and a nurse aide or LPN would be shared between 2 RNs. The nurse manger for this unit was not present, but rather working from home and unavailable for questions or assistance.

A house supervisor was working and available. However, being responsible for the entire hospital, she would not be able to remain on the unit to assist with care. At the time, I was the youngest gatekeeper by years of experience working in this unit. I was not impressed by this change and voiced my concern about the safety of it. There were two other RNs working that day and a full unit of 35 patients. Two nursing assistants split the unit. Together, the three RNs, including myself, completed an unsafe practice report and submitted it to the house supervisor.

Unfortunately, this unsafe practice report did not result in more staff to assist with care. Abandonment of care was not going to be an option, so we went about our day working feverishly to accomplish our tasks and do the best we could for the patients we served. Medications were late, in some cases by over two hours, assessments were not complete, physical care was not complete, the wounds were not properly cared for, documentation was not getting done, and the list went on.

Nearing the end of a 12-hour shift, I had to allow a patient to die alone. For me, this was a turning point in my career and a realization of my responsibility to lead as a gatekeeper in the care of others, regardless of the position I served in, or the level of experience I had, or the risk involved. It broke my heart then and still does today as I reflect on this moment in time.

This patient was restless and calling out, in need of someone to be at his bedside. He had no family. All I could do was run by his room, occasionally stopping to place a hand on his shoulder and encourage his relaxation until he passed away in a fit of fear for what was happening to him. In that moment, I realized that I had to accept the responsibility to take a leadership role, and assure patients received the level and quality care they deserved.

I contacted the Vice President of Nursing due to the absence of my nurse manager requesting an appointment immediately. I was informed by her that she was already home for the day, but that I could come by her home. I assured my patients were handed over to the next shift, contacted the house supervisor asking her permission to clock out for this meeting and to return after to complete my documentation.

The nurses I worked with that day expressed support. However, they also expressed their inability to stand up for what was right because of a fear of retribution and a fear nothing would change. They also expressed that this level of management and leadership was not the responsibility of a staff nurse.

I was also nervous, but regardless, I knew that the right thing to do was to advocate for our patients and our staff and I left to talk with the Vice President of Nursing in her home. Within 24-hours, the model of care shifted and, although not ideal, a team model was put in place, assuring that patient care could be completed as safely as possible.

What I discovered in this situation was that by choosing to do the right thing and serve as a leader, changes occurred in support of those I served. It did not matter that I was the youngest and most novice gatekeeper. I created waves. I was not liked by everyone. I did not lose my job and I did gain respect. Most importantly, however, patients received care.

In ending this chapter, I leave you with our challenge.

Understand that as nurses our profession is only governed by nurses. We have the *power*, and the *responsibility* to be *accountable*, *political* and to practice nursing with *courage* and full authority within our independent as well as collaborative and delegated roles according to our scopes and standards of professional practice. As nurses, we have the obligation to *own* who we are, to *lead*, and to realize our *spiritual* presence, to serve as *gatekeepers*, with full authority to advocate, change health care environments, delegate, develop and implement policy, design and direct delivery of care, communicate, and role model our professional duty, upholding the highest standard in quality and service to others.

Chapter Nine Self-Reflection Challenges

What does being a leader mean to you?

_____

_____

_____

_____

_____

_____

_____

_____

_____

_____

_____

_____

_____

_____

_____

_____

_____

_____

What have you done in your career as a gatekeeper that aligns with your definition of a leader?

_____

_____

_____

_____

_____

_____

_____

_____

_____

_____

_____

_____

_____

_____

_____

_____

_____

_____

What qualities in leadership (visionary, trustworthy, risk taker, etc.) do you demonstrate in your practice as a gatekeeper and how do you demonstrate them?

_____

_____

_____

_____

_____

_____

_____

_____

_____

_____

_____

_____

_____

_____

_____

_____

What can you do today to develop your leadership skills and abilities?

_____

_____

_____

_____

_____

_____

_____

_____

_____

_____

_____

_____

_____

_____

_____

_____

_____

_____

How can you help other gatekeepers develop their leadership skills?

_____

_____

_____

_____

_____

_____

_____

_____

_____

_____

_____

_____

_____

_____

_____

_____

_____

Gatekeepers Create Their Own Future

As gatekeepers, we must create our own future. Nursing by nature is a social profession. Gatekeepers are holistic in assessment and care of not just the person, but groups, and communities as well. Gatekeepers understand the importance of using their skills to support those we care for without judgment. As we look to the future, it is our social nature that assures nursing is the solution to improving access and quality in health care today.

As gatekeepers we are the eyes and ears of the health care community and we know how to utilize our resources to do more with less and to care while maintaining quality and service. Gatekeepers are not supportive of entitlements, but rather supportive of empowering others to take control of their own health care. In order for us to achieve, and sustain this level of influence we must take ownership to tend the gates of health care accordingly and assure that we are present at every bedside, in every clinic, in government, in schools, in businesses, and more. It is our full responsibility to assure that nurses, as the gatekeepers in health care are respected and valued as independent and collaborative partners in that care.

A Call to Serve

In response to the need to examine possible solutions for health care in the United States, the National Academy of Sciences, National Academy of Engineering and the Institute for Medicine (IOM) in collaboration with the Robert Wood Foundation, put together and published a report on nursing. In this report, nursing is recognized as the needed resource for improving access and quality of care (Institute of medicine of the National Academies, 2013). This is positive and recognizes our strength and value as a profession.

As gatekeepers, we must embrace this responsibility and we must lead the way. If not, we will miss the opportunity to serve in our roles as we were meant to serve and will lose significant ground in relation to our independence in practice. It is our responsibility as individual gatekeepers to create our future as a profession. We must not hide behind the image of caring. It is important that we recognize what caring really means and begin to role model it by walking our talk and actively participating in the profession we are.

We must hold ourselves accountable for all actions and non-actions within our profession and in our professional practice. To do nothing, in response to a call for nursing to serve, demonstrates a lack of our own value for who we are and what we can do within our authority as independent and collaborative practitioners. We must accept this challenge and unify as a profession. We must actively demonstrate our value and our responsibility as the gatekeeper in the care of others.

A Moment of Reflection

In chapter three, I shared and example of a chaotic nursing care environment. In this environment nurses were not accepting responsibility and accountability to own their practice independently or collaboratively. As a result physicians became frustrated with the gatekeepers failure to practice according to their professional scopes and standards and by default a medical model of patient care developed. Out of necessity, these physician's, accepted the responsibility to direct the care of every gatekeeper. The care of the gatekeeper became task driven and the goal to complete these tasks verses the goal to achieve positive outcomes became normal routine. These physicians could not trust that gatekeepers caring in this environment were able to manage their independent responsibility.

Ownership of professional nursing practice was being claimed, but not by the gatekeeper. It was claimed by a profession other than the nursing profession. As a result, these physicians did not respect or trust these gatekeepers as collaborative partners in the care of the patients they served. It was not until these gatekeepers accepted ownership of their roles and served with responsibility and accountability to practice to their full potential that these physicians could release the power over the nursing practice of the gatekeepers in this unit and trust that their patients were cared for. When this occurred, census increased, satisfaction increased, turnover decreased, and quality and service scores improved.

Every health care environment is unique. However, the gatekeeper must achieve and maintain authority over their own practice within the scopes and standards of professional nursing practice. Gatekeepers are collaborative and we are independent. Learning to practice prudently in each of these ways is necessary to gain respect as a gatekeeper. By taking this responsibility, nurses claim their future. Nurses then, demonstrate their value from an empowered state, and serve as the leaders they are.

In ending this chapter, and this book, I leave you with the challenge we have been building together. I ask that you reflect on this challenge, maybe tear the page out of this book and place it in a location where you can visualize it daily. Remember, as a gatekeeper you are blessed with the most sacred of all encounters, the human to human relationship. You have been called to serve as the gatekeeper of health care and to ensure safe delivery of care for all in need. This is a great responsibility.

I understand that as nurses our profession is only governed by nurses. We have the *power*, and the *responsibility* to be *accountable, political,* and to *create our future.* We must practice nursing with *courage* and full authority within our independent as well as collaborative and delegated roles according to our scopes and standards of professional practice. As nurses, we have the obligation to *own* who we are, to *lead,* and to realize our *spiritual* presence, to serve as *gatekeepers*, with the full authority to advocate, change health care environments, delegate, develop and implement policy, design and direct delivery of care, communicate, and role model our professional duty, upholding the highest standard in quality and service to others.

Chapter Ten Self-Reflection Challenges

Identify how you can assist the profession of nursing in claiming the future of nursing practice.

_____

_____

_____

_____

_____

_____

_____

_____

_____

_____

_____

_____

_____

_____

_____

_____

_____

_____

How can you as an individual gatekeeper assure that gatekeepers are valued and respected as leaders in health care in your organization and the greater community?

_____

_____

_____

_____

_____

_____

_____

_____

_____

_____

_____

_____

_____

_____

_____

_____

What can you do in your own practice to assure you are in control of your practice and maintaining the nursing scopes and standards of practice?

_____

_____

_____

_____

_____

_____

_____

_____

_____

_____

_____

_____

_____

_____

_____

_____

_____

Reflecting on the content of this book, what has been your greatest take away and why?

_____

_____

_____

_____

_____

_____

_____

_____

_____

_____

_____

_____

_____

_____

_____

_____

_____

_____

_____

References

Bailey, E. (1998). *The new international Webster's pocket dictionary of the English language.* United States: Trident Press International. (p.5)

Blanchard, K.H. (2002). *Whale done!: the power of positive relationships.* New York: Free Press. (p. 113)

Borkowski, S. (2002). *Crying is not an option.* Jackson, MI: S. Lynne Borkowski

Chapman, E. (2005). *Radical loving care: building the healing hospital in America.* Nashville, Tenn: Baptist Healing Trust. (p.93)

Chard, R. The personal and professional impact of the future of nursing report. *AORN Journal,* 273-280. Doi:http//dx.org/10/1016/j.aorn.2013.01.019

Covey, S.M., & Merrill, R. R. (2006). *The speed of trust: the one thing that changes everything.* New York: Free Press. (p.200)

Institute of Medicine of the National Academies (2011). The future of nursing:

leading change, advancing health. National Academies Press. Washington, DC. Retrieved from www.nap.edu

Jenkins, M. & Stewart, A. (2010). The importance of a servant leader orientation. *Health Care Management Review, v35*(1), p. 46-54

Koloroutis, M., editor (2004). *Relationship based care. A model for transforming practice.* Minneapolis, MN: Creative Health Care Management, Inc. (p. 126)

Kunic, R.J. & Jackson, D. (2013). Transforming nursing practice: barriers and solutions. *AORN Journal, v98*(3), p. 235-248. doi:http//dx.doi.org/10.1016/j.aron.2013.07.003

Lynaugh, J. E. (2008). Nursing the great society: The impact of the nurse training act of 1964. *Nursing History Review, 16,* p. 13-28

Macphee, M., Skelton-Green, J. Bouthillette, F., & Suryaprakash, N. (2011). An empowerment framework for nursing leadership development: supporting evidence. *Journal of Advanced Nursing Practice, v68*(1), p. 159-169. doi:10.111/j1365-2648.05746.x

Manion, J. (2005). From management to leadership. Practical strategies for health care leaders. (2nd ed). Sanfrancisco, CA: Jossey-Bass (p. 171)

Marquis, B. L. & Huston, C. J. (2012). *Leadership roles and management functions in nursing.* (7th ed). Philadelphia, PA: Williams and Wilkins (p. 283)

Selenders, L. C. & Crane, P. C. (2012). The voice of Florence Nightingale on advocacy. *Online Journal of Issues in Nursing, v17*(1), p. 1-13. doi:http//dxdoi.org/10.3912/OJIN.Vol17No0 1Man01

Tomey, A. M. (2009). Nursing leadership and management effects work environments. *Journal of Nursing Management, 17*, p. 15-25. doi:10.1111/j.1365-2834.2008.00963.x

Vestal, K. (2010). Designing your own reputation as a leader. *Nurse Leader*, p. 8-10. doi:10.1016/j.mnl/2010/01.010

CPSIA information can be obtained at www.ICGtesting.com
Printed in the USA
LVOW10s0300210716

497185LV00011B/55/P